# A Stroke of Genius

## John M Curcio

## A Stroke/ Healing And Recovery/Life Lessons Meditations

oasisministriersny@yahoo.com

oasisministriesny.org

# DEDICATION

This book is dedicated to all those who have suffered severe injury or illness. It is written to give testimony to the grace of God. It is written so hope may spring into faith and the Lord may encourage the faith of every reader. Our prayer is that the Father will bring healing and health spirit, soul and body.

John M Curcio

# CONTENTS

# Picture Of Area Where Stroke Occurred

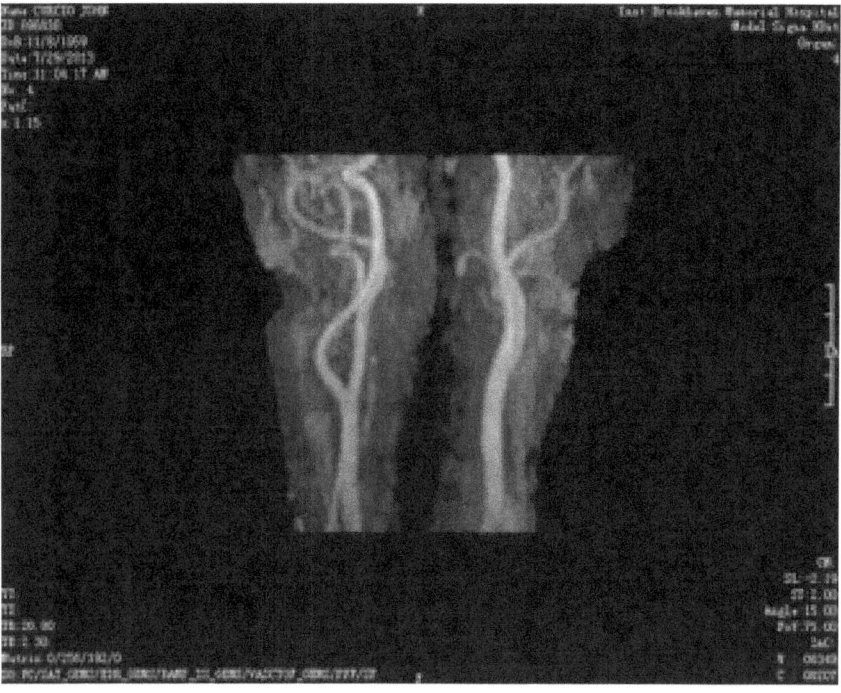

# ACKNOWLEDGMENTS

I would like to thank my wife and family for their support and love. I am also thankful for their constant and helpful insights in the editing and laying out this work. Special thanks for Joe folks an EMT., the Patchogue Ambulance, The Patchogue Fire Department. the beautiful people at Brookhaven Hospital and the wonderful love and prayer support of the Oasis Christian Center family.
Above all else, a special appreciation for our Heavenly Father and the person of His Holy Spirit for inspiration and strength.

All scriptures are taken from either the King James Version or English standard Version of the Holy Scripture

John M Curcio

# Chapter 1.
# Introduction

Eric Cohen wrote an online article about sports entitled,
A New Theory about wrestlers dying young

*Dr. Andrew L. Carney, a Professor at the University of Illinois at Chicago, suspects that the problem wrestlers might be facing is the dissection of the carotid and vertebral arteries in the neck. A dissection happens when a tear occurs in the inner lining of an artery. Because of this, blood enters the space between the inner and outer lining of the artery which then results in the partial or complete blockage of the artery.*
*Dr. Carny's report is revealing.*
*Hyperextending the head or rotating the head aggressively can separate the inner lining of the artery from the outside wall.*

We all face those defining moments in our lives where our lives are changed forever. I had one of those moments. I never expected to face my mortality at 54 years of age. I had my insurances up to date, my beneficiaries in place and certainly was doing my best to exercise. Sometimes our lives are arrested due to a bigger picture. Perhaps we are not seeing something we should be seeing.

Life is made up of so many components. There are physical, spiritual and emotional parts to our lives that make us or break us at times. In these defining moments, we choose to get bitter or better.

In July of 2013 I had a stroke. There is no conclusive evidence that the stroke I had was a sport injury or due to cholesterol and plaque build up. In this testimony, I will include both for the journey. I love football and weightlifting. I could have easily damaged my vertebral artery through contact sports either past or present.

The purpose of this book is to testify of a life altering event and defining moment in my life and my loved ones. I want to give testimony to the grace of God on my life. After having a stroke, I realized the new chapter God had given me in my life. I wanted to accurately recount this journey so those who read may find encouragement and renewed faith in the God of all comfort and love. God bless you in your journey as you read.

# Chapter 2.
# My Journey

I have been fairly healthy all my life. I did have a near death experience as a new born, a strangulated hernia. I also had tonsillectomy and appendix surgery, other than that I have never been hospitalized.

I want to recount the events and circumstances before the stroke. Several factors came into play as I have looked back. It was more like the perfect storm. Hindsight is always 20/20. If we never learn from the past there is a good chance we will repeat it. I have always been health conscious. My last doctor's appointment indicated I needed to lose weight. I also needed to consider cholesterol medicine. The doctor who was himself quite obese, told me to give up pizza. Ouch! That is almost impossible. I enjoyed eating pizza. I did need to address this area but shrugged it off.

There where other areas that may have contributed to my stroke. An overburdened life, an overcharged life and a tendency to overcompensate. I will discuss these issues in the next chapters.

*Whoever conceals his transgressions will not prosper, but he who confesses and forsakes them will obtain mercy. (Proverbs 28:13) ESV*

# Chapter 3 Pre stroke Conditions: Diet / Overweight

I have never had a weight problem but I noticed my waist line growing from a slim 32" to a 40" waistline. I was not fitting into my jeans. To be honest, I always had a bit of a judgmental attitude toward those who were overweight. My journey was unusual because I exercised daily, mostly to develop muscle mass. This technique I learned in my high school and college days. However, as I have gotten older my metabolism has changed. My need for muscle mass is now of less importance than my need for cardiovascular health. I also enjoyed my carbohydrates. I loved my pasta and pizza along with plenty of Italian bread. When I was young, I could eat anything and not gain weight.

As we get older, plaque can builds up around our arteries and create blockages. This may have happened around my vertebral arteries where the stroke occurred. I did not realize I had issues until after the stroke. The last couple of doctor visits revealed that my cholesterol levels were high. My doctor recommended medicine if it did not decline.

I was not moved by his diagnoses. I still ate enough carbohydrates for two people. I was given the name Pasta John as a comical exchange for Pastor John. All that changed after the stroke. I will touch on that in another chapter. I wanted to lay the ground work first. Several issues played into the stroke. Miraculously the stroke did not take my life or leave me disabled.

Losing weight has been very much a journey for me. I did not realize how much of my eating was connected to my emotions. If I was bored, I would snack. If I was upset, I would eat. Most of the eating would be comfort food such as, pasta, breads and such. It is important to make the connections between our emotions and our eating habits. We are told in Scripture not to live by bread alone but by every Word that comes out of the mouth of God.

God permitted the Israelites to go through a season of hunger and leanness so they would learn that life isn't about just food.

*And he humbled you and let you hunger and fed you with manna, which you did not know, nor did your fathers know, that he might make you know that man does not live by bread alone, but man lives by every word that comes from the mouth of the LORD. ( Deut 8:2-3) ESV*

True life is in the Spirit and the Word. The more we allow God to train us to live by His spoken word, the better life gets. Loving God's Word above everything else is the key to freedom. Our emotions can be trained and they must be if we are going to be victorious Christians.

Overcoming emotional eating takes time, effort and concentration. God's grace is sufficient for this. He will help us and empower us to overcome. The more we rely on self-effort alone, the more frustrating it becomes. Each of us are different. God the Father knows best. He can and will show us the best pathway to life and life abundantly in this area of overeating.

*The prudent sees danger and hides himself, but the simple go on and suffer for it. (Proverbs 22:3) ESV*

# Chapter 4. Overburdened

We are told in scripture, to cast our burden on the Lord. Knowing this intellectually is one thing, practicing it is totally different. I have been blessed with good physical strength my whole life. Other than some annoying allergies and sinus conditions, I have been relatively strong and healthy my whole life. Sometimes that can be deceitful. Our strength comes from The Lord. It is when we recognize we are weak in ourselves that we become truly strong.

A series of events were burdening me. I had been concerned for several people. One person was my mother. She was suffering and close to death due to an ulcerated esophagus and other issues. Another was the burden of some people my wife and I pastor. Struggles with drug addiction, financial pressures and marital issues seemed to be hitting many people at once. Another burden was that our church's lease was over and we had to relocate. With all of this happening at once it created the perfect storm of burden and pressure.

*Cast your burden on the Lord, and he will sustain you; he will never permit the righteous to be moved. (Psalm 55:22) ESV*

# Chapter 5. Overcharged

To be overcharged is a little different than being overburdened. They are close cousins. Both can be extremely dangerous to the body. A car battery can be overcharged and die or damage the car. While I am not a car mechanic, it is interesting to note the potential dangers.

*An overcharged battery will boil the sulfuric acid and distilled water mix. The casing of the battery can become hot to the touch, and begin to melt or swell. Flammable hydrogen can build up inside the sealed cells of the battery, causing swelling of the casing under pressure and seepage through small vents. Once the hydrogen is introduced to oxygen, it becomes a sitting time bomb. A small electrical spark can ignite the gas and cause the battery to explode, sending plastic and lead shrapnel flying around, in addition to a caustic sulfuric acid spray. Obviously, this is the most dangerous side-effect of an overcharged battery*
*Jody L Cambell Read more: http:// www.ehow.com/how- does_5137116_happens- overcharge-car-battery.html*

Like a car battery, our lives can be overcharged trying to face the problems of life. We live on the high of what our adrenal glands can provide. The Adrenal gland is available for us to face crisis, tragedy or danger. When we are continually overcharged we are pulling from this source of unusual power. Sometimes way too much. If we continue to operate this way, we will suffer what is called adrenal fatigue, and our bodies can short circuit. I like action. I like being in the middle of it all. Too often, I would tackle things that were not in my grace or my boundary. This requires much more adrenaline.

One of the most common causes of problems in our lives is living outside of our graces or healthy boundaries. Often our pride pushes us over the edge and we break down either physically, spiritually or emotionally. God gives us grace and equips us to handle what is in front of us. We each have a lane to run in. Blessed is the person who finds that lane and stays in it. We will discuss that in a later chapter. Many times in life, we must choose our battles and not feel responsible to solve everyone else's problems. David the king had a great attitude. Something I try to remember.

*O Lord, my heart is not lifted up; my eyes are not raised too high; I do not occupy myself with things too great and too marvelous for me. But I have calmed and quieted my soul, like a weaned child with its mother; like a weaned child is my soul within me. (Psalm 131:1, 2)ESV*

# 6. Overcompensation

How do we overcompensate? We often compare ourselves with others. This is our first mistake. All too often, we recognize and dwell on our weaknesses. We then want to overcompensate. We think that we are not successful in comparison to what others are doing. We try to overcompensate and appear before others as successful to make ourselves feel better.

We also try and overcompensate because our mistakes, poor decisions and misjudgments lead to failures in our lives. We try to overcompensate for the loss. Many times we try to make up for weaknesses in our life by making great sacrifices. This usually leads to disappointment and exhaustion. I have learned something powerful from a man named Ed Cole. Ed Cole had a tremendous ministry to men. A statement which he made has helped me.

*You cannot make up in sacrifice what you have lost through disobedience. Simply obey going forward (Ed Cole)*

# Chapter 7. Staying In Your Grace

When we study the life of Jesus Christ, we see He understood what it meant to stay in one's grace or calling. He was sent to the lost sheep of the House of Israel. If we look at the impact of His life we marvel at a man who stayed in Israel, trained 82 men that we know of for only three years. The impact of the life of Christ Jesus was astounding, considering the limited area in which He worked.

This limitation made the miracle of His life more amazing. No one who ever lived impacted the world like Jesus Christ. We can learn so much from this. He always did what he saw his Father doing. He always said what His Father was saying. Staying in our grace requires humility. H u m i l i t y    i s    n o t weakness. It is knowing our grace gift and calling. It is staying our posts.

I have friends who have traveled the world to minister. They minister to thousands. I have wasted so much time and energy trying to compare or keep up with them. It is all vanity. As I have narrowed down my grace gifts and stay in them, life has greater joy and pleasure.

**He answered, "I was sent only to the lost sheep
of the house of Israel." (Matthew 15:24) ESV**

# Chapter 8. The Stroke

On July 26th, 2013 the journey began. My family and I had been looking forward to vacation the whole year. Every year for the last seven to ten years we have traveled five miles across the Great South Bay to stay at a beach house during the early summer. This particular summer vacation spot is one of our favorite places to go. We were all looking forward to it. This location has been coined the closest place to far away by many Long Islanders. It is truly one of the prettiest places to vacation.

Laurie and I arrived Friday night and loaded everything into the house. As usual, I did not seek any help pushing and loading all our luggage and groceries. By the time I got to the beach house, I was exhausted. We stayed Friday night into Saturday. Saturday other guests began to arrive. We had a wonderful day Saturday at the beach. We enjoyed playing whiffle ball, football and frisbee on the beach. It was just a great time of fun and laughter. We had a wonderful meal for dinner. I went to bed that night knowing that I had to get up early to prepare for Sunday service. I usually go back to the mainland and preach on Sunday and then go back to the beach for the rest of the week.

When Sunday morning came around, I was up as usual around 5am. I went into the living room to read and to pray. I was meditating on Psalm 25 and praying about going back to Long Island. I was a little frustrated because I really wanted to go back Saturday night early so I wouldn't feel rushed. Since moving our church in May and June of 2013, we were in a location with very little storage. Each Sunday we had to set up and take down our equipment. Doing all that was stressful.

As I was reading that morning, I went to stretch lifting up my arms and leaned back. something feelt like it popped. Suddenly, I felt really dizzy like I was about to faint. I fell down to my right side and began to have a pounding headache. I was wondering what was going on. I looked on the Internet for the symptoms for stroke and sure enough I started to see that many of the symptoms I was having were familiar. After that, I then attempted to walk. I wanted to get up to eat or drink something. I found my left side was not responding to my brain's commands. I was dizzy which did not help. I went to the bedroom to lay down as the dizziness continued.

I proceeded to lie down in bed next to Laurie and found my head spinning and getting more dizzy. I asked Laurie to grab two aspirin for me. After she gave me the aspirin, I then began to have the most violent episodes of vomiting I have ever experienced in my life. During that time, I looked out my window and saw Joe Folks a friend of mine who I met at the YMCA. He just "happened" to be walking by and just "happens" to be an emergency medical technician. Joe does not normally come by the house because he doesn't want to seem nosey or intrude on the time that we rent. We rented the house from Joe.

As Joe examined me, he thought initially I had sunstroke. He asked me to touch my nose and to stick out my tongue. He pointed his finger in my eyes to see if they were dilated. He then called the local medical doctor on the island who then came by suburban over to the house. I then walked out to the main wooden walk to meet them. There they drove me to the Davis Park firehouse.

At the firehouse they began to call the police because they saw things that alarmed them. They put me in a wheelchair and wheeled me down to the end of the dock. I was then loaded onto a police boat that had two huge outboard engines. The boat went extremely fast across the water. As they drove across the bay it seem like it was just a moment of time. When we got to the other side, an ambulance was there to meet us by the docks. The EMTs then loaded me onto the ambulance. The gentlemen were so helpful. Since I am a chaplain to the Patchogue fire Department, I know many of the EMTs . One particular fellow who is also a fireman, started joking with me. He said something like this…

**I guess you had a tough time drinking last night.**

I knew he wasn't serious and that he was joking. That is just the way some of the guys are. They know I do not drink. I had all the symptoms of a drunk man. We then drove speedily to the Brookhaven hospital. I was brought to the emergency room and stayed there for most of the morning to early afternoon. They tested me for a virus, heatstroke and such. It all came back negative so they wanted me to stay for further testing. So the following day I had an MRI taken and my primary doctor, Dr. Hill, brought in the laptop computer. Dr. Hill happens to be a believer in Jesus. Several of the interns gathered around my bed as she then told me that I had a major stroke.

She said that I was not equally symptomatic to what the MRI displayed. In other words, I was not showing the symptoms of a stroke of this nature and magnitude. Upon hearing that, I began to weep. You see, I was having one of those why me moments. I was so grateful to God to be alive and get a second chance. She told me that I was

*a walking miracle.*

She also said, knowing that I am a preacher, now you have some really good preaching material.

I went for a few more tests. One of them was a sonogram and while looking at the sonogram of my heart, I said to the technician, it's amazing how God made the body. She replied, yes, that is amazing and I will be believing for your healing from Isaiah 53 which says by his stripes we are healed.

It was nice to know that God had His people set up for me during my time of crisis. God is so good! I was released from the hospital the following Wednesday and went home to recover.

*By His Stripes you were Healed (1Peter 2:24 KJV)*

# Chapter 9. The Healing Journey

I waited three full weeks to go back to the gym to continue my regimen of exercises. Prior to the stroke, I was pushing the envelope with my body by doing some unusual routines with a 18lb. bar. I would roll it around my neck to stretch. Then I would do stair climbing with the bar around my neck. The stroke occurred in my left vertebral artery which is on the back side of my neck. Since the stroke, I have seriously reduced any risk to my neck. At present, I am doing much more cardio exercises than I had previously done. It had taken a good three weeks to regain my confidence in the gym. Initially, I was afraid to drive, workout and afraid to swim for fear I would drop dead or something. One day I was driving to a speaking engagement. I was about three miles away. I suddenly had a panic attack that felt like the stroke symptoms returning. I called Dr. Hill and she said, it was just nerves and to put on some worship music to calm down.

Wow! Imagine that. I am sure she could have prescribed some drug but she knew what I needed.

*If you will diligently listen to the voice of the LORD your God, and do that which is right in his eyes, and give ear to his commandments and keep all his statutes, I will put none of the diseases on you that I put on the Egyptians, for I am the LORD, your healer.(Exodus 15:26)*

# Chapter 10. The Neurologist

When I left the hospital, one of the doctors on duty recommended for me to see a doctor at Stony Brook Hospital. Several people told me that Dr. Woo was one of the best neurologists in the world. While I was waiting for him in the examination room, the Word of The Lord came to me. Now if you have ever had that happen you, you know it is not just a result of mental memorization. Memorization is a healthy practice. I recommend it highly. Memorization and meditation played a significant role in my healing. The Last chapter of this book gives some helpful advise and verses for meditation. However, this experience came more like an authoritative voice.

*And it shall come to pass in that day, [that] his burden shall be taken away from off thy shoulder, and his yoke from off thy neck, and the yoke shall be destroyed because of the anointing.(Isaiah 10:27) KJV*

The key words were, *Yoke off thy neck.* Dr. Woo

went on to explain where the blockage was. It was in the vertebral artery in the back of my neck. I was elevated in my faith as the Word of The Lord confirmed what Dr. Woo was to say to me.

I love the Word on healing more than I love healing. I love the Word on prosperity more than I love prosperity. I love the Word! While I deeply respect Dr. Woo, I felt the diagnosis from heaven was all I needed.

*Remove your stroke from me;*
*I am spent by the hostility of your hand. (Psalm 39:10 ESV)*

# 11. Giving Credit Where Credit Is Due

It is important to express deep gratitude for all the things that God has done, is doing and is going to do in our lives. It is also important to express gratitude to all the people who play an important role in our miracles. I would like to touch on as many of them as possible.

First of all, I would like to express my gratitude to God and the redemptive work of Christ. Without whom I can do nothing. I thank God for His Holy Word. His Word has been my anchor through many a crisis. This was no exception. I looked to God for a good word at every stage of healing and recovery. The Lord is the strength of my life. When I am the weakest, I am the strongest.

Secondly, I must mention how my wife acted so courageously. It takes a lot of courage to hold it together while your husband has a stroke. She was watching the symptoms take hold as she rode with me to the hospital. I also am not the best patient to deal with. I was a cranky patient. A person like myself who is always going here and there, always busy with something, is hard to tie down. I needed to rest! While home for three weeks, I was not the most pleasant company. We have to be careful not to take out our frustrations on those closest to us, but often we do. My wife gets an extra jewel in her crown for patience and long suffering.

My children and Laurie all filled in while I was off for two weeks from church duties. My son John filled in one week and Laurie filled in the other. I am so proud of them both. I love David and Grace. I know they were deeply concerned. They helped in every way they could. I am blessed with an awesome family. My mom, my sister Debbie and her husband Tony came to visit in the hospital. Again, I am blessed. My brother Steve and Kathy called and I knew I had their prayers as well. Tony actually lent me a pair of shorts while in the hospital. For some reason, he had two pairs of shorts on. He literally took the shorts off his butt and gave them to me!

Next, I thank the praying church. I am the person people are always calling for prayer. Now I needed it. I have learned to never underestimate the power of prayer. We should all be connected in some way to a group or team of people who know how to pray. It is more important than health, life or fire insurance. While I recommend Insurance, to neglect prayer ministry is foolish.

I have had a wonderful opportunity to be the Chaplain for the Patchogue Fire Department. I have tried to be there for them in their times of need for about 23 years now. I have come to admire and appreciate these men and women who serve our communities. Particularly the volunteers. Many of the firemen and women also serve in the local ambulance company. I have always admired what they do. When I needed them most they were there in perfect timing and excellent service. The local police were there in such a hurry and were so awesome in their response to this incident. We need to keep these men and woman in our prayers and when given the opportunity express deep appreciation.

**Render therefore to all their dues: tribute to whom tribute is due; custom to whom custom; fear to whom fear; honor to whom honor. (Romans 13:7) KJV**

# Chapter 12. Exercise

I have developed a habit of exercise over the years. While the credit to a quick recovery cannot be given totally to exercise, I believe it is important to appreciate the role exercise plays in overall health.

As I said in an earlier chapter, I was trained to build muscle mass due to the type of sports I played. I thought that was being masculine. Since then, I realized how futile that is later in life. My exercise routine has incorporated more cardio. I was introduced to life of exercise through my older brother Steve. I love and respect Steven. He is eight years older than I am. I always looked up to him and his skills in sports. He played an important role in my life especially after my dad died in 1970. I was ten years old then.

My mom always exercised regularly and worked with senior citizens helping them exercise. I believe the disciplines gained through sports and exercise helped me recover quicker. I remember going in to my MRI. I was very bored. I began an exercise routine in my hospital bed. I would do simple things like leg lifts and arm lifts. I was leaning towards physical therapy before I felt the call of God on my life towards ministry. I purposely put exercise last as far as credit goes. So much emphasis is put on the outer body today. The spirit of man is often neglected.

*The spirit of a man will sustain his infirmity (Proverbs 18:14) KJV*

The apostle Paul recognized the benefits of exercise. He also made it very clear that Godly living was the highest benefit to man's wellbeing.

*While bodily training is of some value, godliness is of value in every way, as it holds promise for the present life and also for the life to come. (1Timothy 4:8)ESV*

# Chapter 13. Coming Home

As I stated before, I was not the easiest patient. After two days I wanted to escape. I told the doctor I was getting cranky and just wanted to go home. My wife deserves a medal of service award for putting up with me. All the nurses, doctors and technicians were awesome. They all did their best to encourage me to stay for all the tests they felt I needed. I am glad I stayed. Miraculously, I was discharged Wednesday afternoon. I felt like Jonah. Three days in the belly of the whale. Many lessons can be learned in the belly of a whale. After coming home I had three weeks of recovery before I could get back into the swing of things. Many people showed their support by stopping by the house.

You realize how many beautiful people there are that love you when you need them the most. I got a bit frustrated about my new diet. I cheated one day and had my daughter Grace go out to a local burger place for a huge burger.

On the way home, Grace got into a car accident. I felt so bad about that. Fortunately she was physically fine. That was a six hundred dollar hamburger! The car repair cost $600.00!

Emotionally, it was very draining for her and Laurie. I ended up doing my best to fix her car. She later had gotten a beautiful Jeep that she loved. I am so proud of everyone that helped. I felt caged in being home for three weeks of recovery. Needless to say, I was cranky. I made it more stressful on Laurie. The three weeks seemed like an eternity

*Bear one another's burdens, and so fulfill the law of Christ. (Gal 6:2) ESV*

# Chapter 14. Be True To Yourself

I always thought the statement "be true to yourself" was a corny statement. I realized after the stroke how important it was. Often, when we repress our true feelings about things, they will eventually surface some other way. That was the case with me. Once you have a near death experience, you realize how short and fragile life is. For me, I began to speak my mind more freely with others. It was quite evident with my family. I also became less soft spoken. For better or worse a new person had arrived. I just could not stuff anymore.

I do not believe it is healthy to stuff. We must find ways to express how we feel when we disagree with others or others hurt us or aggravate us. Some people will not like the new you, but trying to be liked by everyone is so laborious and dangerous. It can wear your mind, body and spirit out. To be true to yourself does not mean we have to be rude or unloving. It does mean we must be honest. We live in a world where political correctness is the eleventh commandment. People are losing their jobs over speaking their minds. We must be free to speak out when we disagree with something. We must be free to be angry. We must control the anger if it leads to sin. While we can and should love all men, we do not have to embrace their lifestyle. Satan works in the arena of half-truths and lies. He is also the champion of strife, uncontrolled anger and wrath. As believers, we are free to be angry. Anger without self-control is the devil's playground.

Meekness is part of the fruit of the spirit. Meekness means power under control. When we speak truth it must be seasoned with grace. Jesus did not come with grace only. He came with grace and truth. Grace and truth must both work together to experience freedom. We are so afraid to address sin as sin, abuse as abuse, immorality as immorality for fear of being politically incorrect. Sometimes we love our reputation before men more than truth. God help us.

*Therefore, having put away falsehood, let each one of you speak the truth with his neighbor, for we are members one of another. 26 Be angry and do not sin; do not let the sun go down on your anger, 27and give no opportunity to the devil.*
*(Ephesians 4:25) ESV*

# 15. D-Stressing

I was told by my doctor to pick up a blood pressure machine. I try to use it as often as I can. It can be stressful in itself. I realized I needed to keep my blood pressure as normal as possible by d-stressing. How do I d-stress? Of course prayer, forgiveness, quiet meditation are essential. It is also important to stay contrite and humble while being as quick to forgive as we can.

One day, I was taking my blood pressure and someone was telling me a joke. I laughed so hard. I noticed my blood pressure showed normal levels. I thought that was Interesting. A happy heart is good medicine just like proverbs says.

Part of d-stressing is making sure we choose our battles. Not every crisis is ours to be concerned about. Somewhere in our spiritual training we feel we have to carry the world's burdens. Each of us have a passion for something. Whatever our passion is, is usually the problem that we are called to help solve or bring healing to. It is when we go beyond that grace in our life, that we fail and frustrate the grace of God on our lives. God's grace is on us and in us to serve and bless God in worship and to serve one another with our varied gifts and talents.

*A merry heart does good like a medicine (Proverbs 17:22) KJV*

# Chapter 16. Delegate

This is a bit hard to admit, but I have struggled with delegating responsibilities to others. It is from a root of pride and lack of faith in God and others. Delegating is a great way to mentor and build relationships. I am glad I am not alone in this. Moses the great prophet of God also fell into this trap. Let's look at the story in Exodus.

*The next day Moses sat to judge the people, and the people stood around Moses from morning till evening. When Moses' father-in-law saw all that he was doing for the people, he said, "What is this that you are doing for the people? Why do you sit alone, and all the people stand around you from morning till evening?" And Moses said to his father-in-law, "Because the people come to me to inquire of God; when they have a dispute, they come to me and I decide between one person and another, and I make them know the statutes of God and his laws." Moses' father-in-law said to him, "What you are doing is not good. You and the people with you will certainly wear yourselves out, for the thing is too heavy for you. You are not able to do it alone. Now obey my voice; I will give you advice, and God be with you! You shall represent the people before God and bring their cases to God, and you shall warn them about the statutes and the laws, and make them know the way in which they must walk and what they must do. Moreover, look for able men from all the people, men who fear God, who are trustworthy and hate a bribe, and place such men over the people as chiefs of thousands, of hundreds, of fifties, and of tens. And let them judge the people at all times. Every great matter they shall bring to you, but any small matter they shall decide themselves. So it will be easier for you, and they will bear the burden with you. If you do this, God will direct you, you will be able to endure, and all this people also will go to their place in peace." So Moses listened to the voice of his father-in- law and did all that he had said. Moses chose able men out of all Israel and made them heads over the people, chiefs of thousands, of hundreds, of fifties, and of tens. And they judged the people at all times. Any hard case they brought to Moses, but any small matter they decided themselves. Then Moses let his father-in-law depart, and he went away to his own country. (Exodus 18:13-27) ESV*

As you can see, Moses listened to the advice of his

Father-in law. Advice from the right people can save our lives. I love Psalm one. It says, that a man is blessed when he does not walk in the council of the ungodly. I was not always quick to get advice. I hated the feeling of not knowing. Now I simply ask for help. If I do not understand what someone is saying I will ask for help. I may say, please forgive my ignorance in this. Please explain.

I was always afraid to ask questions in school. I suffered needlessly due to fear and pride. It usually takes a time in our life where we are reduced to nothing that we begin to value good advice and help from others.

We should not wait until we are reduced to nothing. We should be quick to admit we do not know it all and you cannot do it all. That is when God's grace comes in and things are easier. Humility is a wonderful posture. It is not thinking less of ourselves. It is admitting we can do nothing without Christ. It is also the confidence that we can do all things through Christ who strengthens us.

*I can do all things through Christ who strengthens me (Philippians 4:13) KJV*

# Chapter 17. Closing Lessons

In closing, I would like to encourage us all. It has been said that hindsight is always 20/20. I have officiated quite a few funerals in my day. When we have a near death experience, we tend to count every day precious and every person as valuable and precious.

I will often tell those attending a wake service to reflect personally and try to live each day more passionately. I would often say, love more deeply, laugh more loudly and forgive more frequently. I also would remind us all to live in the present. The word present has two meanings. It means live in the now and live in the gift. Each day is a gift. Live in the present!

*NOW Faith is (Hebrews 11:1) KJV*

# Chapter 18 The Power Of Meditation

The word meditate carries the meaning to mutter or to speak softly. Often, people equate meditation to some eastern religious cult. In reality, the practice of meditation is an ancient practice of the Hebrews.

In our culture today, our society is becoming more acquainted with the word meditation with the modern yoga movement. However, this can be deceptive as yoga is tied to the hindu religion. The Hindu religion boasts of about 500 million gods. That is right, 500 million with an M. Just because we may disagree with the Hindu faith, we ought not disregard the practice of meditation. Yoga and it's varied positions are connected indirectly to the worship of some deity other than Christ.

I know Scriptural centered meditation works. Meditation can lead us to a healthier, life, wealthier life and more joy in our relationship with God and others.

Keep in mind, as you practice this wonderful art, that thoughts produce beliefs, beliefs produce words, words produce life or death. Depending on the results you want, healthy, purposeful meditation can lead to a more fruitful life.

Below are some verses of scripture on healing. Practice reciting them slowly from the heart. Memorize if you want. It is more important to assimilate these truths in the heart than accumulate info in the brain.

When we eat natural foods, they start out as plant or animal life. These foods then become digested and assimilated into our blood stream to distribute nutrients to our entire body. In the same way, scripture when assimilated, distribute life to the body, mind and spirit. Remember to give praise and make it personal while in the process of meditation. Say it like this, I thank you Lord that I ...... whatever verse you are quoting. This is very important in the process. Gratitude releases tremendous faith and power.

Enjoy!!!


*Study this Book of Instruction continually. Meditate on it day and night so you will be sure to obey everything written in it. Only then will you prosper and succeed in all you do. Jos 1:8 NLT*

*But they delight in the law of the LORD, meditating on it day and night. Psa 1:2 NLT*

*My child, pay attention to what I say.*
*Listen carefully to my words. Don't lose sight of them.*
*Let them penetrate deep into your heart, for they bring*
*life to those who find them, and healing to their whole*
*body. Guard your heart above all else,*
*for it determines the course of your life. Pro 4:20-23*
*NLT*

*O LORD my God, I cried unto thee, and thou hast*
*healed me. Psalm 30:2 (KJV)*

*Let all that I am praise the LORD;*
*may I never forget the good things he does for me.*
*He forgives all my sins*
*and heals all my diseases.*
*He redeems me from death*
*and crowns me with love and tender mercies.*
*He fills my life with good things.*
*My youth is renewed like the eagle's! NLT*

*He sent his word, and healed them, and delivered*
*[them] from their destructions.Psalm 107:20 (KJV)*

*But he [was] wounded for our transgressions, [he was]*
*bruised for our iniquities: the chastisement of our*
*peace [was] upon him; and with his stripes we are*
*healed. Isaiah 53:5 (KJV)*

*Heal me, O LORD, and I shall be healed; save me,*
*and I shall be saved: for thou [art] my praise.*
*Jeremiah 17:14 (KJV)*

*Then said he unto me, These waters issue out toward the east country, and go down into the desert, and go into the sea: [which being] brought forth into the sea, the waters shall be healed. Ezekiel 47:8 (KJV)*

*The diseased have ye not strengthened, neither have ye healed that which was sick, neither have ye bound up [that which was] broken, neither have ye brought again that which was driven away, neither have ye sought that which was lost; but with force and with cruelty have ye ruled them. Ezekiel 34:4 (KJV)*

*And his fame went throughout all Syria: and they brought unto him all sick people that were taken with divers diseases and torments, and those which were possessed with devils, and those which were lunatick, and those that had the palsy; and he healed them. Matthew 4:24 (KJV)*

*The centurion answered and said, Lord, I am not worthy that thou shouldest come under my roof: but speak the word only, and my servant shall be healed. Matthew 8:8 (KJV)*

*When the even was come, they brought unto him many that were possessed with devils: and he cast out the spirits with [his] word, and healed all that were sick: Matthew 8:16 (KJV)*

*And Jesus went forth, and saw a great multitude, and was moved with compassion toward them, and he healed their sick. Matthew 14:14 (KJV)*

*And great multitudes followed him; and he healed them there. Matthew 19:2 (KJV)*

*And he healed many that were sick of divers diseases, and cast out many devils; and suffered not the devils to speak, because they knew him.Mark 1:34 (KJV)*

*For he had healed many; insomuch that they pressed upon him for to touch him, as many as had plagues. Mark 3:10 (KJV)*

*And they cast out many devils, and anointed with oil many that were sick, and healed [them].*
*Mark 6:13 (KJV)*

*But so much the more went there a fame abroad of him: and great multitudes came together to hear, and to be healed by him of their infirmities.Luke 5:15 (KJV)*

*And the whole multitude sought to touch him: for there went virtue out of him, and healed [them] all. Luke 6:19 (KJV)*

*And when the woman saw that she was not hid, she came trembling, and falling down before him, she declared unto him before all the people for what cause she had touched him, and how she was healed immediately. Luke 8:47 (KJV)*

*And they held their peace. And he took [him], and healed him, and let him go; Luke 14:4 (KJV)*

*And Jesus answered and said, Suffer ye thus far. And he touched his ear, and healed him. Luke 22:51 (KJV)*

*There came also a multitude [out] of the cities round about unto Jerusalem, bringing sick folks, and them which were vexed with unclean spirits: and they were healed every one. Acts 5:16 (KJV)*

*For unclean spirits, crying with loud voice, came out of many that were possessed [with them]: and many taken with palsies, and that were lame, were healed. Acts 8:7 (KJV)*

*Confess [your] faults one to another, and pray one for another, that ye may be healed. The effectual fervent prayer of a righteous man avails much. James 5:16 (KJV)*

*Who his own self bare our sins in his own body on the tree, that we, being dead to sins, should live unto righteousness: by whose stripes ye were healed. 1 Peter 2:24 (KJV)*

*He sent his word, and healed them, and delivered*

*[them] from their destructions.Psalm 107:20 (KJV)*

*O LORD my God, I cried unto thee, and thou hast healed me. Psalm 30:2 (KJV)*

# A Prayer For You

May the Lord the Healer touch you at the point of your need. May you experience his unfailing love cover your spirit, soul and body; may the multidimensional love of the Father fill your heart; may the grace of the Lord Jesus Christ touch every fabric of your being and may the fellowship of the Holy Spirit guide you throughout your life. In Jesus' name amen!

Salvation Prayer
Heavenly Father I come to You, just as I am, asking for the gift of eternal life in Jesus Christ. I declare Jesus as Lord and believe He has risen from the dead. I turn from my ways to follow Your ways. Thank you for the amazing gift do eternal life. Thank you that my sins are forgiven and that Heaven is my home. In Jesus' name, Amen

## ABOUT THE AUTHOR

Pastor John Curcio is married to his wife Laurie for 37 years. Together after John attended Oral Roberts University, they attended Rhema Bible Training College. Upon graduation, they returned to New York to seek God's will for their lives. In 1993, Oasis Ministries was born and they have been serving as Pastors for 24 years. John has also served as Chaplain to the Patchogue Fire Department for 21 years. Pastors John and Laurie have 3 grown children and two grand children. Together with his wife and children, they have composed dozens of original songs and Pastors John and Laurie have authored 12 books.

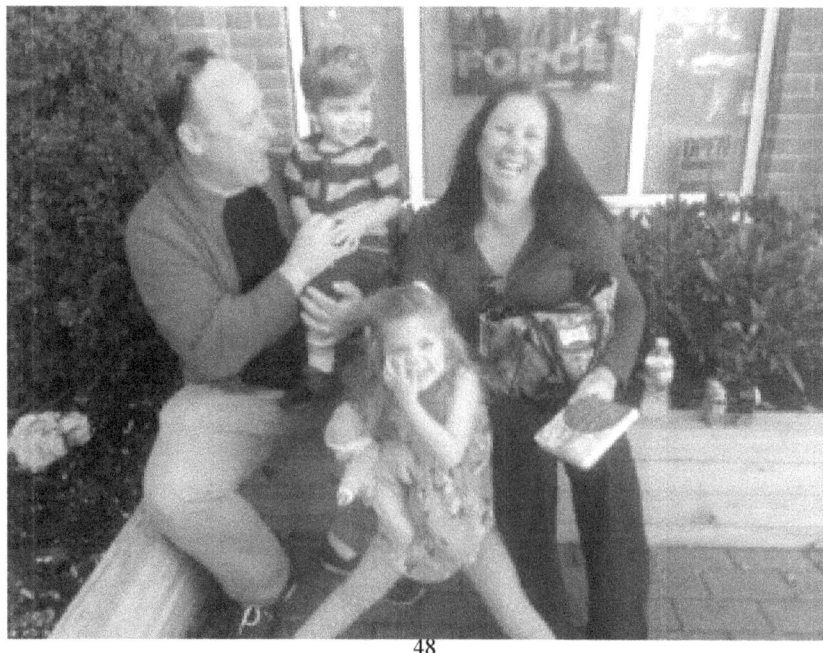